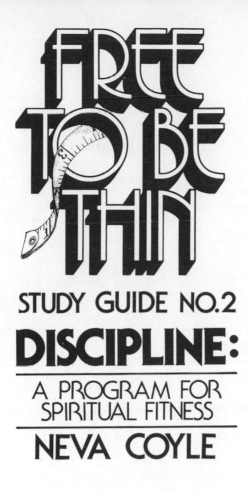

STUDY GUIDE NO. 2

DISCIPLINE:

A PROGRAM FOR SPIRITUAL FITNESS

NEVA COYLE

Do you not know that those who run in a race all run, but only one receives the prize? Run in such a way that you may win.

And everyone who competes in the games experiences self-control in all things. They then do it to receive a perishable wreath, but we an imperishable.

Therefore I run in such a way, as not without aim; I box in such a way, as not beating the air; but I buffet my body and make it my slave, lest possibly, after I have preached to others, I myself should be disqualified.

I Corinthians 9:24-27

Study II in OVEREATERS VICTORIOUS program for Christian weight loss.

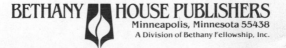

BETHANY HOUSE PUBLISHERS
Minneapolis, Minnesota 55438
A Division of Bethany Fellowship, Inc.

A NOTE FROM NEVA

I welcome you to this second series to help you reach your desired goal weight. Many OV'ers have stated that this series is their favorite. During this series you will be looking at the principle of a disciplined life and the work God wants to do in you through discipline and the purpose of it all. I pray a special blessing of insight and understanding for you as you now begin this study.

Because of Jesus,

Neva Coyle

Free To Be Thin Study Guide No. 2—
Discipline
Neva Coyle

Copyright © 1980
Neva Coyle
All Rights Reserved

Published by Bethany House Publishers
6820 Auto Club Road, Minneapolis, Minnesota 55438

Printed in the United States of America

Books by Neva Coyle:

Free To Be Thin, w/Marie Chapian, a successful weight-loss plan which links learning how to eat with how to live

There's More To Being Thin Than Being Thin, w/Marie Chapian, focusing on the valuable lessons learned on the *journey* to being thin

Slimming Down and Growing Up, w/Marie Chapian, applying the "Free To Be Thin" principles to kids

Living Free, her personal testimony

Daily Thoughts on Living Free, a devotional

Scriptures for Living Free, a counter-top display book of Scriptures to accompany the devotional

Free To Be Thin Cookbook, a collection of tasty, nutritious recipes complete with the calorie content of each

Free To Be Thin Leader's Kit, a step-by-step guide for organizing and leading an Overeaters Victorious group, including five cassette tapes of instruction

Free To Be Thin Daily Planner, a three-month planner for recording daily thoughts, activities and calorie intake

BEFORE YOU BEGIN

There are special Journal Sheets that have been assigned Bible readings to be used along with your study for each week.

LESSON ONE

For Your Preparation—Basic Journal Sheet

1ST DAY _____ TIME ____ REFERENCE: I Tim. 4:7; II Peter 1:1-2, Rom. 1:1-7

God is impressing on me: | I've shared with the Lord . . .

Thoughts I'm having today: _____

_____

_____

2ND DAY _____ TIME ____ REFERENCE: II Peter 1:3, I Peter 1:3-9

God is impressing on me: | I've shared with the Lord . . .

Thoughts I'm having today: _____

_____

_____

3RD DAY _____ TIME ____ REFERENCE: II Peter 1:4, Eph. 4.11-16

God is impressing on me: | I've shared with the Lord . . .

Thoughts I'm having today: _____

_____

_____

4TH DAY _____ TIME ____ REFERENCE: II Peter 1:5-8, John 17

God is impressing on me: | I've shared with the Lord . . .

Thoughts I'm having today: _____

_____

_____

5TH DAY _____ TIME _____ REFERENCE: II Peter 1:9; I John 1:5-10, 2:1-2

God is impressing on me: | I've shared with the Lord . . .

Thoughts I'm having today: _____

_____

_____

6TH DAY _____ TIME _____ REFERENCE: II Peter 1:10; Rom. 11:29; Matt.

God is impressing on me: | 22:14; II Thess. 2:13-15; Jude 24
I've shared with the Lord . . .

Thoughts I'm having today: _____

_____

_____

7TH DAY _____ TIME _____ REFERENCE: II Peter 1:1-10

God is impressing on me: | I've shared with the Lord . . .

Thoughts I'm having today: _____

_____

_____

_____

WEEKLY EVALUATION

What principles has the Lord taught me this week? _____

_____

How can I be more faithful in honoring the Lord next week? _____

_____

What changes am I seeing in my attitude towards:

Food? _____

God? _____

Others? _____

SPIRITUAL EXERCISES

Read II Peter 1:1-10

In the Amplified Version of the Bible, we find such interesting insights and new perspectives. It is with the determination to find out all that God has to say to us that we find it most helpful to read in various translations.

II Peter 1:1

> "Simon Peter, a servant and apostle (special messenger) of Jesus Christ to those who have received (obtained an equal privilege of) like precious faith with ourselves in and through the righteousness of our God and Savior Jesus Christ."

This verse is for us to recognize who the whole book of II Peter is written to.

"To those who: _____

_____

Who are these? _____

Does that include you? ———— How do you know? _____

_____

II Peter 1:2

> "May grace (God's favor) and peace (which is perfect well-being, all necessary good, all spiritual prosperity and freedom from fears and agitating passions and moral conflicts,) be multiplied to you in (the full, personal, precise and correct) knowledge of God and of Jesus our Lord."

According to this verse from the Amplified Bible, define:

Grace: _____

_____

Peace: _____

_____

As overeaters we can be assured of many implications of this verse. We can be freed from the fear of:

(Check the ones that apply in your life.)

____ Not getting enough to eat.

____ Getting sick because of dieting.

____ Not reaching the goal.

____ Looking too gaunt when reaching goal.

____ Being full of pride when reaching goal.

(Name other specific fears you have.)

_____

_____

We can be freed from the agitating passions of:
(Check those that apply to you.)

____ Outrageous appetites

____ Non-stop eating

____ Eating out of anger

____ Eating when depressed

____ Eating when lonely

____ Eating when feelings are hurt

____ Eating when frustrated or tired

____ Eating because of boredom

(Name other specific agitations you have known.)

_____

_____

_____

II Peter 1:3

"For His divine power has bestowed upon us all things that (are requisite and suited) to life and godliness, through the (full personal) knowledge of Him who called us by and to His own glory and excellence (virtue.)"

Whose power? _____ *"He _____ bestowed."*

PAST TENSE! ALREADY GIVEN!

For what kind of life? _____

Through what? _____

What does that mean to you when you are faced with temptations of food? _____

_____

_____

_____

II Peter 1:4

"By means of these (His divine power and the knowledge of Him) *He has bestowed upon us His precious and exceeding great promises so hat through them you,* _____ _____ (your name), *may escape (by fligh from the moral decay."*

Look at that phrase *"by flight."* Indicated here is the pov r to turn from temptations with food and walk away. Leave the kitchen. Put the lid or the cookie jar and leave the room! Escape! Unharmed and still intact with the program and with God, even more victorious than before. It is a way into victory. You now have good reason to praise God. A way of escape through His power and a knowledge of Him. He supplies all we need.

II Peter 1:5

"For this very reason (verse 4), adding to your diligence (to the divine promises) employ every effort in exercising your faith to develop virtue (excellence, resolution, Christian energy), and in (exercising) virtue (develop) knowledge (intelligence)."

Define the following:

Virtue: _____

_____

Resolution: _____

_____

Christian energy: _____

_____

Knowledge: _____

_____

The beginning of your spiritual exercise program starts with warm-ups like a physical exercise program (which, by the way, you should begin to pray about). For your warm-ups you have been diligent in the Word!

II Peter 1:6

> *"And in exercising knowledge develop self-control, and in exercising self-control develop steadfastness (patience, endurance), and in exercising steadfastness develop godliness (piety)."*

Define "exercise": _____

_____

Define "self-control": _____

_____

How do you exercise self-control? _____

_____

Define "steadfastness": _____

_____

How does one exercise steadfastness? _____

When exercised, what does steadfastness develop? _____

Define "godliness": _____

_____

II Peter 1:7

> *"And in exercising godliness develop brotherly affection, and in exercising brotherly affection develop Christian love."*

How does one exercise godliness? _____

_____

Define "brotherly affection": _____

_____

How does one exercise brotherly affection? _____

_____

Define "Christian love": _____

_____

Many of us try our best to operate in the realm of brotherly love and Christian love without first spending time in the Word. We try our best to love others without first spending time exercising our virtue. Have you ever tried to do a hundred sit-ups without any previous exercise program? It is doubtful that anyone could do 25 sit-ups, let alone 100. Well, that is exactly what it is like in the spiritual realm to try to give brotherly love and develop Christian love without the first of the warm-up and shape-up exercises. Many ask, "But isn't that selfish, spending time building myself up?" No! It isn't! It is essential for you in order to give out genuine Christian love. DO NOT get the cart before the horse in the spiritual exercise program. These exercises are essential in your everyday walk in the Spirit.

I Peter 1:8

> *"For as these qualities are yours and* increasingly *abound in you, they will keep you from being idle or unfruitful unto the full personal knowledge of our Lord Jesus Christ, the Messiah, the Anointed One."*

These qualities are to be _____ in our lives.

They will keep you from being _____ or _____ unto the full personal knowledge of _____.

Do you need that? _____

II Peter 1:9

> *"For whoever lacks these qualities is blind, spiritually shortsighted, seeing only what is near to him, and has become oblivious of the fact that he was cleansed from his old sins."*

What happens when a person doesn't do these exercises? _____

_____

What happens to those who do not realize they are cleansed from their old sins? _____

_____

II Peter 1:10

> *"Because of this, brethren, be all the more solicitous and eager to make sure (ratify, to strengthen, to make steadfast) your calling and election, for if you do this you will never stumble or fall."*

What is your calling and election? _____

_____

For further thought, read Romans 12.

How do you ratify and strengthen your calling? _____

_____

YOU, _____, WILL NEVER STUMBLE OR FALL!
     (your name)

10

Review these exercises!
1. Limber up—diligence in the Word.
2. Stretch—exercise your faith.

"Faith cometh by hearing and hearing by the Word of God." Romans 10:17

3. Trimmers and tighteners:
   —virtue
   —knowledge
   —self-control
   —steadfastness (long-suffering)
   —godliness
   —brotherly affection
   —Christian love

BE SPIRITUALLY FIT!

ASSIGNMENT:

1. Have a daily quiet time, using the Basic Journal Sheet. It will help you prepare for each week's lesson. Read and record other scriptures in your Journal.
2. Stay within your calorie limit.
3. Commit yourself to being someone's spiritual support partner in prayer. Exchange phone numbers and call them this week when prompted by the Holy Spirit.
4. Review Chapters 6 and 18, *Free To Be Thin*, by Marie Chapian.
5. Now go on to Lesson Two, using the Basic Journal Sheet as a daily guide for preparation.

For Your Preparation—Basic Journal Sheet

1ST DAY _____ TIME _____ REFERENCE: I Cor. 10:13

God is impressing on me: | I've shared with the Lord . . .

Thoughts I'm having today: _____

2ND DAY _____ TIME _____ REFERENCE: Heb. 12:1-3

God is impressing on me: | I've shared with the Lord . . .

Thoughts I'm having today: _____

3RD DAY _____ TIME _____ REFERENCE: Matt. 26:36-40, 56

God is impressing on me: | I've shared with the Lord . . .

Thoughts I'm having today: _____

4TH DAY _____ TIME _____ REFERENCE: Matt. 26:41-50

God is impressing on me: | I've shared with the Lord . . .

Thoughts I'm having today: _____

5TH DAY _____ TIME ___ REFERENCE: Matt. 26:67-75

God is impressing on me: I've shared with the Lord . . .

Thoughts I'm having today: _____

_____

_____

6TH DAY _____ TIME ___ REFERENCE: Matt. 27:26-31

God is impressing on me: I've shared with the Lord . . .

Thoughts I'm having today: _____

_____

_____

7TH DAY _____ TIME ___ REFERENCE: Matt. 27:35

God is impressing on me: I've shared with the Lord . . .

Thoughts I'm having today: _____

_____

_____

WEEKLY EVALUATION

What principles has the Lord taught me this week? _____

How can I be more faithful in honoring the Lord next week? _____

What changes am I seeing in my attitude towards:

    Food? _____

    God?_____

    Others? _____

GOD'S PROVISION FOR ENDURANCE

I Corinthians 10:13 (AMP)

"For no temptation—no trial regarded as enticing to sin (no matter how it comes or where it leads)—has overtaken you and laid hold on you that is not common to man—that is, no temptation or trial has come to you that is beyond human resistance and that is not adjusted and adapted and belonging to human experience, and such as man can bear. But God is faithful (to His Word and to His compassionate nature), and He (can be trusted) not to let you be tempted and tried and assayed beyond your ability and strength of resistance and power to endure, but with the temptation He will (always) also provide the way out—the means of escape to a landing place—that you may be capable and strong and powerful patiently to bear up under it.

Study Hebrews 12:1-3.

1. What are the sins that cling so close?

_____

_____

Did you include overeating?

OVEREATING IS A WORKING OUT OF SOMETHING GOING ON INSIDE. WHAT?

_____

_____

_____

What is the race God has set before you (verse 1)? _____

_____

How many calories per day? _____

2. ENDURANCE. Look to _____ the author and perfector of our faith. You can see that we are not expected to have perfect faith from the beginning. "Perfector" indicates an ongoing, changing, progressing process.

When we look to one thing, we are looking away from something else. In our eating habits, when we look to Jesus for help and support, we look _____ from food.
And when we look at food, we look _____ from Jesus.

3. ENCOURAGEMENT. When thinking of the opposition and bitter hostility Jesus faced, what comes to mind? Look at Matthew.

a. Matt. 26:36-40, 56 _____

b. Matt. 26:41-50 _____

c. Matt. 26:67 _____

d. Matt. 26:69-75 _____

e. Matt. 27:26 _____

f. Matt. 27:28-31 _____

g. Matt. 27:35 _____

We are considering what Jesus went through in comparison to the trials we are going through. Why? _____

_____

THIS COMPARISON IS NOT MEANT TO SHAME US OR TO PUT US UNDER CONDEMNATION FOR FEELING LOW IN THE TIME OF TRIAL, BUT RATHER TO POINT OUT TO US THAT WE HAVE A SAVIOR IN JESUS WHO KNOWS HOW WE FEEL. WE ARE TO BE ENCOURAGED BY HIS EXAMPLE AND FOLLOW IT.

ASSIGNMENT:

1. Read and record scripture daily in your journal.
2. Stay within your calorie limit, keep a calorie account sheet.
3. Call your OV prayer partner or friend this week when the Holy Spirit prompts you, when you are in need or when you can encourage your partner.
4. Prepare Lesson 3.
5. Read Chapter 8, *Free To Be Thin*, by Marie Chapian.
6. Project: List the areas of your life that are disciplined. Then make another list of the areas of your life that are not so disciplined. Ask the Lord to show you how to bring discipline into the unruly areas of your life.

For Your Preparation—Basic Journal Sheet

1ST DAY _____ TIME ____ REFERENCE: Heb. 12:5-8
God is impressing on me: | I've shared with the Lord . . .

Thoughts I'm having today: _____

2ND DAY _____ TIME ____ REFERENCE: II Tim. 3:16-17
God is impressing on me: | I've shared with the Lord . . .

Thoughts I'm having today: _____

3RD DAY _____ TIME ____ REFERENCE: Heb. 12:9-11
God is impressing on me: | I've shared with the Lord . . .

Thoughts I'm having today: _____

4TH DAY _____ TIME ____ REFERENCE: Psalm 119:71
God is impressing on me: | I've shared with the Lord . . .

Thoughts I'm having today: _____

5TH DAY _____ TIME ____ REFERENCE: Heb. 12:12-14

God is impressing on me: | I've shared with the Lord . . .

Thoughts I'm having today: _____

_____

_____

6TH DAY _____ TIME ____ REFERENCE: Rom. 13:14

God is impressing on me: | I've shared with the Lord . . .

Thoughts I'm having today: _____

_____

_____

7TH DAY _____ TIME ____ REFERENCE: I Cor. 9:24

God is impressing on me: | I've shared with the Lord . . ,

Thoughts I'm having today: _____

_____

_____

WEEKLY EVALUATION

What principles has the Lord taught me this week? _____

_____

How can I be more faithful in honoring the Lord next week? _____

_____

What changes am I seeing in my attitude towards:

Food? _____

God?_____

Others? _____

DISCIPLINE AND CORRECTION

Hebrews 12:5, 7 (AMP)

> "*And have you [completely] forgotten the divine word of appeal and encouragement in which you are reasoned with and addressed as sons? My son, do not think lightly or scorn to submit to the correction and discipline of the Lord, nor lose courage and give up and faint when you are reproved or corrected by Him. You must submit to and endure correction for discipline. God is dealing with you as with sons, for what son is there whom his father does not thus train and correct and discipline?*"

Study: Hebrews 12:5-14.

Vs. 5. We are told that we have been addressed as _____. We are not to think lightly or to scorn to submit to the _____ or _____ of the Lord. Neither are we to _____ or _____ or _____ when we are _____ or corrected by Him.

Vs. 6. If the Lord is correcting you in any area, not just eating, it proves He _____ you.

Vs. 7. Do we have any choice in the matter of correction or discipline of the Lord in our lives? _____

Vs. 8. What about those who want to be exempt from correction? _____
_____

Vs. 9. In the Living Bible and in the Amplified Version, it says not only to submit to the Father in discipline, but to do it cheerfully. Is that easy? _____ Is it impossible? _____

Vs. 10. Why does God discipline us? _____
_____

Can we now see the truth in Psalm 119:71? _____
_____

Vs. 11. Does it say that we will like the discipline? _____ What is the discipline in your own life that you are experiencing right now? _____
_____
_____
_____

What does the discipline yield? _____
_____

"Conformity to God's will in purpose (obedience), *thought (setting our minds) and action* (submission)."

Vs. 12. So now what are we going to do? Are we to have great pity parties for ourselves, complete with refreshments? Hate all the thin people? Hold unforgiveness toward those who try to get us to eat when they know we are retraining our eating habits? Should we resist counting calories as a silent protest? What are we supposed to do?

Paraphrase verse 12 to apply to yourself: _____

_____

_____

_____

Vs. 13. How are we going to make firm and straight and plain and smooth paths for our feet?

Apply this truth to your eating program: _____

_____

_____

Vs. 14. Are we at peace with everyone when we are overeating? _____ Are we at peace with everyone when we grudgingly stay on our program? _____ *"Pursue that consecration and holiness without which no one will ever see the Lord."* How do we pursue consecration and holiness? _____

_____

_____

_____

ASSIGNMENT:

1. Continue in journal and daily scripture reading.
2. Account for calories eaten daily, recording them on your sheet.
3. Study Hebrews 12:14-29.
4. Read Chapter 10, *Free To Be Thin*, by Marie Chapian.
5. Prepare yourself in prayer and then ask your mate (if married) how your being in OV affects him/her.
6. Call an OV friend at least once this week.

NOTE:

Have you ordered the next series? Now would be a good time if you plan to go on. Use the form in the back of the book to receive a current price list.

For Your Preparation—Basic Journal Sheet

1ST DAY _____ TIME ____ REFERENCE: Heb. 12:14-17; Ecc. 4:9-12

God is impressing on me: | I've shared with the Lord . . .

- -

Thoughts I'm having today: _____

_____

_____

2ND DAY _____ TIME ____ REFERENCE: Gen. 25:29-34

God is impressing on me: | I've shared with the Lord . . .

- -

Thoughts I'm having today: _____

_____

_____

3RD DAY _____ TIME ____ REFERENCE: I Pet. 1:23; I John 3:9, 4:7, 5:1-4, 18

God is impressing on me: | I've shared with the Lord . . .

- -

Thoughts I'm having today: _____

_____

_____

4TH DAY _____ TIME ____ REFERENCE: Heb. 12:18-24

God is impressing on me: | I've shared with the Lord . . .

- -

Thoughts I'm having today: _____

_____

_____

5TH DAY _____ TIME _____ REFERENCE: Rom. 14:4, Ps. 91:11, I Cor. 12:25-27;
God is impressing on me: I John 1:9, Heb. 12:1, Gal. 5:1
                                                    I've shared with the Lord . . .

- -

Thoughts I'm having today: _____
_____
_____

6TH DAY _____ TIME _____ REFERENCE: Heb. 12:25-29
God is impressing on me: I've shared with the Lord . . .

- -

Thoughts I'm having today: _____
_____
_____

7TH DAY _____ TIME _____ REFERENCE: Ex. 19:5, 23:20-22; I Sam. 15:22; Jer.
God is impressing on me: 7:23-24
                                                    I've shared with the Lord . . .

- -

Thoughts I'm having today: _____
_____
_____
_____

WEEKLY EVALUATION

What principles has the Lord taught me this week? _____
_____

How can I be more faithful in honoring the Lord next week? _____
_____

What changes am I seeing in my attitude towards:
   Food? _____
   God? _____
   Others? _____

21

STRENGTHENING THROUGH DISCIPLINE

Study: Hebrews 12:14-19

Vs. 14. Define "strive": _____

_____

Review how we pursue consecration and holiness from the last lesson. _____

_____

_____

Vs. 15. How can you exercise forethought in your eating plan?

_____

_____

_____

We are encouraged in this passage to look after one another. How can we do that in OV?
(Read Ecc. 4:9-12): _____

_____

_____

Vs. 16-17. Have you ever felt like Esau felt after you have eaten something you know you
shouldn't?_____ Read Genesis 25:29-34. What is a birthright? Look in the dictionary
for some ideas. _____

_____

_____

What is our birthright as born-again Christians?

    I Peter 1:23 _____

    I John 3:9 _____

    I John 4:7 _____

    I John 5:1-4 _____

    I John 5:18 _____

How does that knowledge help you in your eating plan? _____

_____

_____

_____

The difference between Esau and us is that we can find repentance from our transgression through confession and forgiveness in Jesus Christ (I John 1:9).

Vs. 18–21. We are not approaching a physical kingdom that causes us to tremble in fear of death.

Vs. 22–24. Rather we come unafraid to a spiritual kingdom, to God who provided the way to himself through Jesus Christ. Listed in these verses we find all the defenses we ever need at our disposal. They are:

The Living God (Romans 14:4) _____

Angels (Psalm 91:11) _____

The Church (I Cor. 12:25-27) _____

The Judging God (I John 1:9) _____

The Redeemed in Heaven (Heb. 12:1) _____

Jesus (Galatians 5:1) _____

Vs. 25. Why is it important that we accept His correction and teaching and learn to obey Him?

Exodus 19:5 _____

Exodus 23:20-22 _____

I Samuel 15:22 _____

Jeremiah 7:23 _____

Other favorite scriptures:

_____   _____

_____   _____

_____   _____

Vs. 27. Is God shaking your eating habits? _____

Is God shaking your will? _____

Is God getting your attention through your battle with food? _____

If God shakes you up in this area of your life, what is the "unshakeable" that will remain when He is through? _____

_____

_____

_____

Vs. 28. When we come through this "shaking up," what will we be able to offer God? __

_____

_____

_____

Define "godliness": _____

_____

_____

_____

Compare your definition with the answer to the previous question. _____

_____

_____

Vs. 29. What is a consuming fire? _____

_____

Apply that to our relationship with God: _____

_____

_____

_____

ASSIGNMENT:

1. Continue in your journal—recording daily scripture reading, new teachings the Lord reveals to you, new insights in understanding yourself, areas where the Lord is disciplining you.
2. Account for the calories you eat by recording them on your Calorie Account Sheet. Stay within your limit.
3. Exercse forethought in your eating plan at least three consecutive days this week.
4. In keeping with verse 15 of Hebrews 12, call an OV friend at least twice this week.
5. List the ways you can "strive" to live in peace.
   a. With yourself:

   b. With your mate:

   c. With your family:

   d. With others who are important in your life:

7. Read Chapter 15, *Free To Be Thin*, by Marie Chapian.
8. Prepare for Lesson 5. Use the Basic Journal Sheet to help you in preparation and study.
9. Continue with your physical exercise program.

For Your Preparation—Basic Journal Sheet

1ST DAY _____ TIME ____ REFERENCE: Rom. 8:6

God is impressing on me: | I've shared with the Lord . . .

Thoughts I'm having today: _____

_____

2ND DAY _____ TIME ____ REFERENCE: Rom. 7:22-23

God is impressing on me: | I've shared with the Lord . . .

Thoughts I'm having today: _____

_____

3RD DAY _____ TIME ____ REFERENCE: Philippians 4:7-8

God is impressing on me: | I've shared with the Lord . . .

Thoughts I'm having today: _____

_____

4TH DAY _____ TIME ____ REFERENCE: Eph. 4:22-24

God is impressing on me: | I've shared with the Lord . . .

Thoughts I'm having today: _____

_____

_____

5TH DAY _____ TIME _____ REFERENCE: Eph. 4:25-32
God is impressing on me: I've shared with the Lord . . .

- -

Thoughts I'm having today: _____

_____

_____

6TH DAY _____ TIME _____ REFERENCE: Luke 9:23
God is impressing on me: I've shared with the Lord . . .

- -

Thoughts I'm having today: _____

_____

_____

7TH DAY _____ TIME _____ REFERENCE: Eph. 6:10–18
God is impressing on me: I've shared with the Lord . . .

- -

Thoughts I'm having today: _____

_____

_____

_____

WEEKLY EVALUATION

What principles has the Lord taught me this week? _____

_____

How can I be more faithful in honoring the Lord next week? _____

_____

What changes am I seeing in my attitude towards:
- Food? _____
- God? _____
- Others? _____

DISCIPLINING THE MIND

WE NEED TO DISCIPLINE OUR MINDS:

Romans 8:6 (NAS)

"For the mind set on the flesh is _____ but the mind set on the Spirit is _____ and _____."

Romans 7:22-23. What are the three laws listed here?

1. The law of _____ in my _____

2. The law of my _____ in my _____

3. The law of _____ in my _____

Two of these laws war against each other. Which laws are these?

_____ vs _____

IF OUR MINDS WERE SET ON THE SPIRIT (Romans 8:6), THEN OUR MINDS WOULD BE IN HARMONY WITH THE "LAW OF GOD IN THE INNER MAN" AND WE COULD THEN CONTROL THE "LAW OF SIN IN THE MEMBERS OF YOUR BODY." THEN GOD PROMISES US PEACE.

Philippians 4:7 (NAS):

"And the _____ of God, which surpasses all comprehension shall _____ your _____ and _____ in Christ Jesus."

Ephesians 4:22-24:

Vs. 22. We are told: _____ lay _____ the _____ self, which is being _____."

Vs. 24: "Put on the _____ self, which in the likeness of God has been created in _____ and in the holiness of the _____."

Verse 23 tells us how to get from verse 22 to verse 24. How is that? "Be _____ in the _____ _____ _____ _____."

WE NEED A CHANGE IN OUR WAY OF THINKING!
WE NEED DISCIPLINE OF THE MIND THROUGH RENEWAL . . .

There follows in this chapter of Ephesians a check list of things we can do to bring about this renewed mind or changed thinking. Check the items that you need to deal with in your life:

___ Lay aside falsehood and speak truth.

___ Deal with angry feelings immediately.

___ Don't give the devil any opportunity.

___ Behavioral reform.

___ Launder conversation.

___ Don't grieve the Holy Spirit.

___ Bitterness, unresolved discord in your life or relationship.

___ Be more kind to others.

___ Unforgiveness.

THE CARNAL MIND DOES NOT ADHERE TO THE SCRIPTURAL MIND BY ITSELF—WE NEED DISCIPLINE!

Philippians 4:7-8

We need to censor what goes into our minds to find a place there.

TEN PRINCIPLES THAT LEAD US TOWARD A DISCIPLINED THOUGHT LIFE:

1. Become aware of God's power in your life:
   —place yourself daily in God's hands.
   —don't go in your own strength.
2. Consult with God about your life each day. Moment by moment, learn to walk in the Lord.
3. Don't let your mind become careless or slack.
4. Refuse to look at the past with regret—but to the future with faith.
5. Feed on the Word of God.
6. Pray without ceasing. Praise. Be diligent in communion with God.
7. Walk in the light of obedience.
8. Resist the devil with all spiritual weapons available to you. Do not ever treat mental oppression or condemnation as one of those "natural" things.
9. Deal quickly with failure.
10. If the enemy breaks through, stand firm. Don't let him have any more ground. Then call your OV friend or prayer partner.

ASSIGNMENT:

1. Review lessons on Discipline. Make a list of things you learned and relate how it has helped you in your eating plan.
2. Have a daily quiet time. Record in your journal the scripture you have read and what the Lord is teaching you.
3. Account for the calories you have eaten each day.
4. Call an OV friend or prayer partner this week.
5. Set a goal for the week.
6. Read Chapter 16, *Free To Be Thin*, by Marie Chapian.

CALORIE ACCOUNT SHEET (Sample)

NAME _____ WEEK OF _____ TO _____

Week's Beginning Weight _____ Calorie Limit _____ Starting Weight _____ Goal Weight _____ Week's Ending Weight _____

	1st Day Portion	1st Day Cal.	2nd Day Portion	2nd Day Cal.	3rd Day Portion	3rd Day Cal.	4th Day Portion	4th Day Cal.	5th Day Portion	5th Day Cal.	6th Day Portion	6th Day Cal.	7th Day Portion	7th Day Cal.
MORNING														
total														
MIDDAY														
total														
EVENING														
total														
Daily total														

Tape Albums and Study Guides by Neva Coyle:

(The study guides come with the tape albums but may also be ordered separately.)

A Seminar on Living Free (four cassettes) A recording of her seminar in which she shares the principles that have helped her break free from a life of misery and self-satisfaction
Living Free Study Guide, to accompany the tape album

Free To Be Thin (seven cassettes) Victory, Weight-loss, Deliverance
Free To Be Thin Study Guide No. 1, Getting Started, to be used with the book by the same title, and/or the tape album

Discipline (four cassettes) A Program for Spiritual Fitness
Free To Be Thin Study Guide No. 2, Discipline, to be used with the book by the same title, and/or the tape album

Abiding (four cassettes) Honesty in Relationships
Abiding Study Guide

Freedom (four cassettes) Escape from the Ordinary
Freedom Study Guide

Diligence (four cassettes) Overcoming Discouragement
Diligence Study Guide

Obedience (four cassettes) Developing a Listening Heart
Obedience Study Guide

Free To Be Thin Aerobics, available in LP record album with booklet, or cassette tape album with booklet

Restoration (three cassettes) Helping restore those who may have faltered in their spiritual life or commitment
Restoration Study Guide

Perseverance (four cassettes) For People Under Pressure
Perseverance Study Guide

Detach here

For information regarding OVEREATERS VICTORIOUS and for current price lists on other materials, send a business-size, stamped, self-addressed envelope to Overeaters Victorious, Inc., P.O. Box 179, Redlands, CA 92373.

If you would like to receive special mailings concerning Overeaters Victorious seminars in your area, fill out the form below. (*Allow four weeks.*)

Please print or type

Name _____

Address _____

City/State _____ Zip _____